One is all, all is one.

We and the others are the same.

Thinking about the others is thinking about ourselves.

Taking care of the others is taking care of ourselves.

Aphorism of Prof. Bui Quoc Chau

Titolo | Dien Chan - First Aid
Autore | Truong Thi My Le
ISBN | 978-88-27823-38-5

Youcanprint Self-Publishing
Via Roma, 73 - 73039 Tricase (LE) - Italy
www.youcanprint.it
info@youcanprint.it
Facebook: facebook.com/youcanprint.it
Twitter: twitter.com/youcanprintit

Dedicated to all children and all teenagers, especially those of the elementary courses of "Dien Chan for Children", who gave me the motivation to start and complete this work. I wish them to be the pebble in the pond that will widen more and more the wave hoops.

Dedicated to all grandparents and parents, who may benefit from it in their daily life and help their children and grandchildren to strengthen their ability to self-healing

Dedicated to my daughters, nieces and nephews, hoping they may always be proud of having two cultures and hoping they may use both to be helpful to humanity.

Acknowledgments

I would like to thank prof. Bui Quoc Chau for sharing his discoveries, experience, teaching and for his continuous search for beauty and simplicity.

I would like to thank all vietnamese reflexologists, who reported and shared their experience over time, first of all prof. Tran Dung Thang, the eldest student of prof. Bui Quoc Chau. Thanks to his collection of "1001 tricks of Dien Chan" I started to write this booklet.

I thank my family for the patience and collaboration during the long work of reading, translating, writing and drawing.

I thank my daughter Elizabeth for the picture of the lady's face and the various pictures of the hands.
I thank my sister Duyen who always supports me in my plans even when they are too ambitious and optimistic.
I thank all the people who are trying to spread this wonderful technique; my brother Tri in first place who pursues the goal of training more reflexologists and trainers.
Finally I thank you for forgiving any imperfections in this work.

INTRODUCTION

"Dien Chan - Vietnamese multi-reflexology facial" is a
method born in 1980 in Ho Chi Minh city (Viet Nam),
thanks to the studies and experiments of prof. **Bui Quoc
Chau** and his collaborators.

*It is a method that allows people to recover or maintain
good health without resorting to the use of medicines,
scalpels and needles but simply by massaging, pressing,
tapping or heating certain points on the face, or parts of the
body, which reflect the organs or areas of dysfunction.*

*It is a natural therapy that aims to restore the energy
balance of the body, stimulating a response from the latter,
through reflex points.*

- It's simple

- It's effective

- It's cheap

- It can also be done with fingers or knuckles

- It can be done anytime and anywhere

*Finally, it is a technique that allows anyone to become
aware of the state of their health, to intervene at the first
symptoms of illness and to support their body during
classical medical treatments, accelerating their recovery
time.*

*This booklet collects Dien Chan treatments that can help in
some of the most common emergency situations.*

This is not all that can be done for these inconveniences, but emergency interventions that could allow us to get quickly out of it.

They are simple massages derived from Dien Chan's theories, its reflex maps, its reflex points and its similarities of form, which do not pretend to replace the official First Aid but to relieve it from less serious situations, so that it can concentrate on the most important ones.

The elaboration of this collection is based on the successful experiences of Vietnamese reflexologists who have been practicing this method for over 30 years, as well as on direct experiences of the author and of the people who she has been able to suggest these massages to.

All the massages reported in the collection can be done with bare hands or with means almost available everywhere (water, hair dryer ...), so that they can be practiced by everyone and in any situation. Who has learnt more about Dien Chan, however, knows that its founder, prof. Bui Quoc Chau, while claiming that all the massages can be done with the tools that we all always have at hand, the fingers, he has invented, together with his sons and son-in-law, more than 130 instruments, so that everyone can have what he likes more and adapt it, in order to obtain better results with less effort. In the book, therefore, there are some suggestions that involve the use of some Dien

Chan tools, in order to permit those in possession of them to obtain even more surprising results.

Try it to believe.
But believe in what?
In ourselves, first and foremost.
Once you have experienced that you can actually cure yourself with simple massages, you will realize that you are really strong and that the body is a small miracle from a loving Creator: he gave everyone a car and also everything needed to repair it if it fails.

The work is intended for everyone, so even for those who still have to approach Dien Chan and his theories, adults and even children. Everyone can take advantage of it as long as they want to get involved.

I hope I have done a useful job and have contributed to realize the dream of prof. Bui Quoc Chau, that is

TRANSFORM THE PATIENT
IN
DOCTOR OF HIMSELF

Good health to everyone and, please, try these treatments because, as prof. Bui says, it's a bet where, if you win, you will feel better and if you do not win, nothing changes.
Truong Thi My Le

INSTRUMENTS

Stressing that, to practice the massages proposed here, the bare hands are more than enough, since I mentioned the use of some particular tools and means, I report a brief description here, so that people who do not know them can have an idea of them.

DOUBLE RAKE

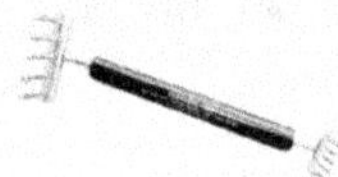

Length: 14 cm
Weight: 26 g
Material: plastic and stainless steel

The small rake is used on the areas reflected on the face, especially along the eyebrows to relax the shoulders and neck pains, while the large one is used to stimulate the scalp and for the treatments that refer to the diagram of the human body on the head. It is a very useful tool on people with signs of stress, nervousness or depression. Its use for a few minutes is sufficient to relax and eliminate the headache; regulates the nourishing functions of the scalp and helps to reduce hair loss, dandruff and fat.

FINDER - TOOTHED BRASS ROLL

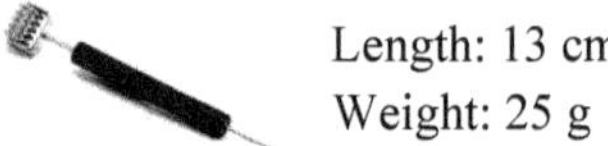

Length: 13 cm
Weight: 25 g
Material: plastic, stainless steel and brass

It is one of the basic tools; at one end it carries a notched brass roller and at the other a stainless steel rounded point. The tips are all rounded. The metal roller cylinder allows to lower the body temperature. It is used when we are facing an excess of heat, such as fever, prolonged exposure to sunlight, itching, burns, various inflammations, etc. The stainless steel point makes it possible to identify reflex points and to stimulate them with greater precision.

TOOTHED PLASTIC ROLL AND SMOOTH BRASS BALL

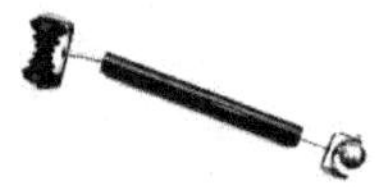

Length: 14 cm
Weight: 26 g
Material: plastic and stainless steel

Very complete tool: the smooth sphere is used to relax the tensions of the eye, liver and digestive system. Its consistency and its material provide Yin effects (relaxing, refreshing, dispersing). It is also used on the hands and fingers to relieve joint pain. The Yang concave roller is suitable for massaging the toes, eyebrows, neck and jaw.

ROLLER WITH STEEL NEEDLES

Length: 13 cm

Weight: 16 g

Material: plastic and stainless steel

The roller of this instrument is equipped with stainless steel tips that stimulate the activation of the superficial microcirculation of the skin. It disperses heat and helps to rebalance the body in cases of sudden changes in temperature. It gives excellent results on couperose, on expression wrinkles, water retention in the eye contour and is recommended before applying cosmetics.

BIG DOUBLE PLASTIC BALL

Length: 18 cm

Weight: 170 g

Material: plastic and stainless steel

It is a Yang type instrument with spheres of about 3 cm that allow you to work on larger areas of the body (back, stomach, legs, arms, shoulders, buttocks). It is a powerful activator of blood circulation; stimulates and relaxes at the same time; warms the cold areas of the body, it is also very effective in the treatment of cellulite and the elimination of fat, with a simple massage lasting 5-6 minutes each day on the affected area.

MOXA

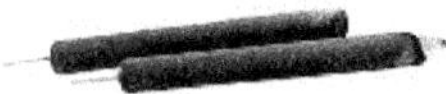

Moxa is an instrument that derives from acupuncture, it is used to stimulate the reflex zones of the affected parts through heat.

It is a cigar made of a mixture of medical herbs in which Artemisia predominates, a shrub with numerous medicinal properties including:

• Antiseptic (property to prevent or slow down the development of microbes);

• Antispasmodic (reduces muscle spasms and also relaxes the nervous system);

• Diaphoretic (facilitates skin transpiration);

• Expectorant (favors the expulsion of bronchial secretions);

• Eupeptic (promotes digestion).

The use of moxa is very effective in the stimulation of reflex points, in the treatment of joint pain, sinusitis and otitis. This use, however, must be limited and carried out by reflexologists who have good knowledge of Dien Chan techniques.

HEATING BALSAM

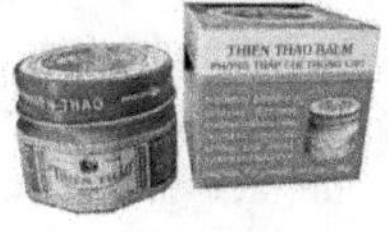

it is used to heat the contracted areas due to the cold or to grease the reflex points or areas to be stimulated. Very little is needed at the tip of the search points, or finger, to feel the effect. On the market there are several types, the best known is the Tiger balsam, but any warming balm can be used, provided it does not create irritation to the skin.

HEATING PATCHES

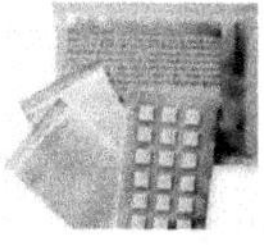

They are patches of camphor and menthol, common in the market to treat muscle pains, especially used by athletes. In Dien Chan they are used in the form of small 4 mm square stamps, to be applied on the reflex points, or 1 cm to be applied on the areas to be stimulated, to have a stimulation with the heat that they release, for a period of about 2 hours.

There are different brands and sizes, but prof. Bui Quoc Chau, after many tests, considers those of the Salonpas brand to be the most effective.

POINTS

In some cases, points with their respective numbers have also been highlighted. For those who do not know it, Dien Chan starts from the discovery that on our face there are points that reflect the whole body, comparable to medicinal plants, each with specific effects and therapeutic indications.

These points have been baptized by Prof. Bui Quoc Chau with numbers. About 1000 points have been discovered on the face, but currently around 600 are used, of which only about fifty are really used.

The points given here are intended only to remind those who already know the method, the importance of some of them, and their usefulness in various emergency situations.

Who wants, then, can act directly on the points indicated to get results faster, those who still do not know them yet or at the moment can not find them precisely, do not worry, just act on the areas indicated.

I hope these clarifications have been helpful. I repeat, I could have completely avoided mentioning these technical details, but I thought that this small work will also be in the hands of people who already have a certain knowledge and some tools and that with it they could use even better what they have.

ACHILLES' HEEL

Heat with the hair dryer, or press the exact point of the pain on the heel of the other foot for a few minutes. If necessary, repeat several times.

Massage the upper part of the neck, with the fingertips of the fingers or, better still, with the knuckles of the index and the middle fingers.

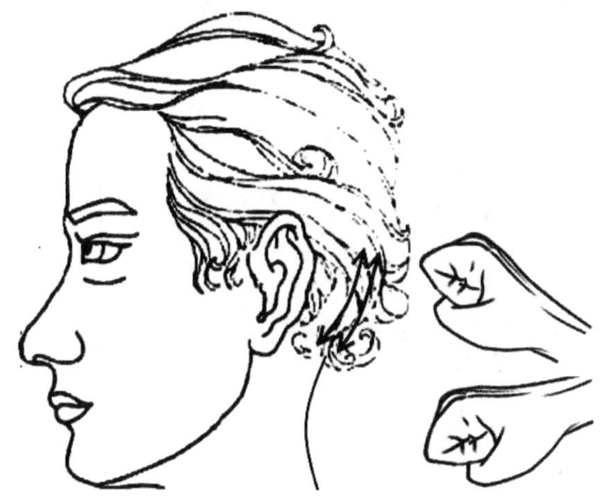

ANKLE - INFLAMMATION DISTORTION

Heat the wrist of the injured ankle with a hairdryer (or moxa) for 2 or 3 minutes. Repeat several times a day if the problem persists.

Otherwise you can rotate the same wrist 30-50 times and massage along the wrinkle of the chin, insisting on the most painful areas.

WARNING: AVOID CHIN MASSAGE IF YOU ARE PREGNANT

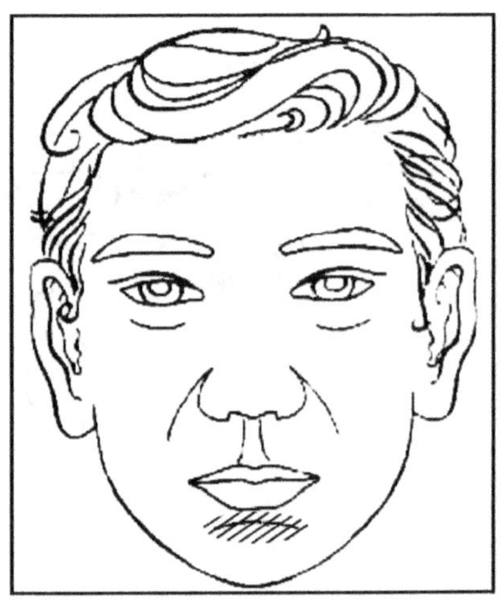

[14]

ASMA ATTACK

As soon as the crisis begins, actively stimulate the point at the base of the nose, between the nostrils (point 19) for about 1-2 minutes, then, with the thumbs fingertips, massage the sides of the nose, with circulatory movements, outwards of the cheeks.

(point 19 is at the base of the nose, press it with your finger at about 45 °)

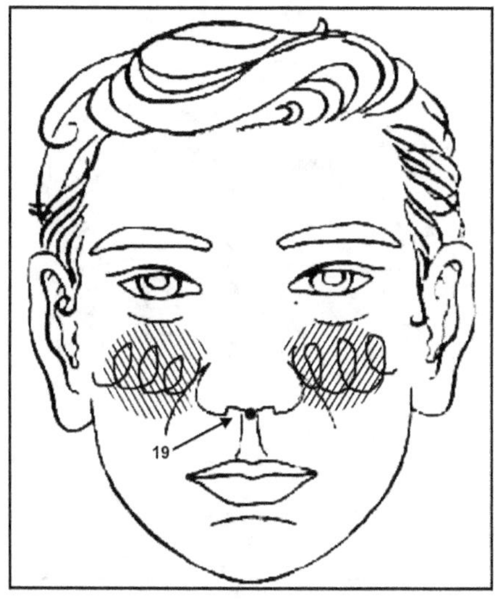

BACKACHE

Massage with the knuckles of the fingers, backwards, or tap with the fingertips, the dotted areas, with a tolerable pressure; where there is a more painful point, insist more (about 1 minute).

If you have a Dien Chan roll, you can roll on the same areas In addition, scrape the scalp, with the fingers a little bit bent (or the rake of Dien Chan), from the front to the zenith, for 30-50 times. Where you feel more pain, scrape for several times

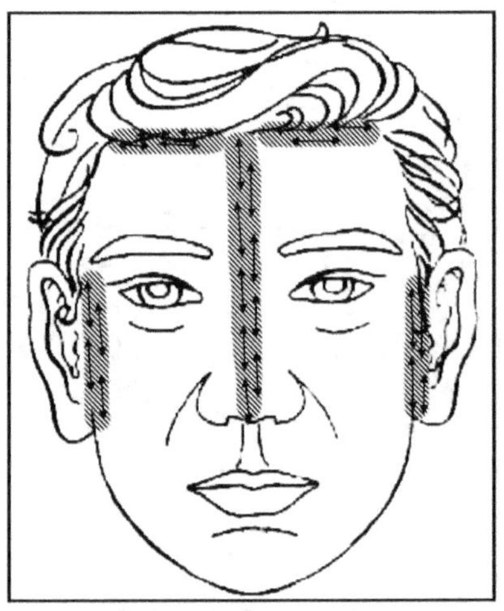

BITTER MOUTH

Tap strongly the indentation under the lower lip, where there is point 235, for 20-30 times.

WARNING: **DO NOT PRACTICE THIS MASSAGE IN CASE OF PREGNANCY**

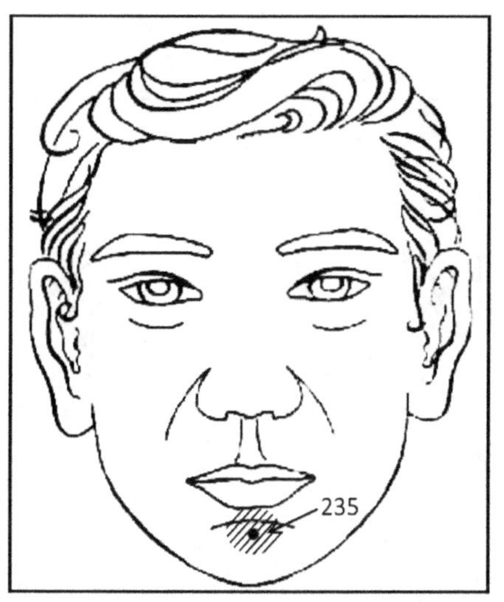

BREATH (BE OUT OF)

Massage with the three middle fingers, from top to bottom, with a certain pressure, the area of the beginning and between the two eyebrows (for about 1-2 minutes). WARNING: this massage can lead to a rapid lowering of blood pressure in individuals sensitive to hypotension

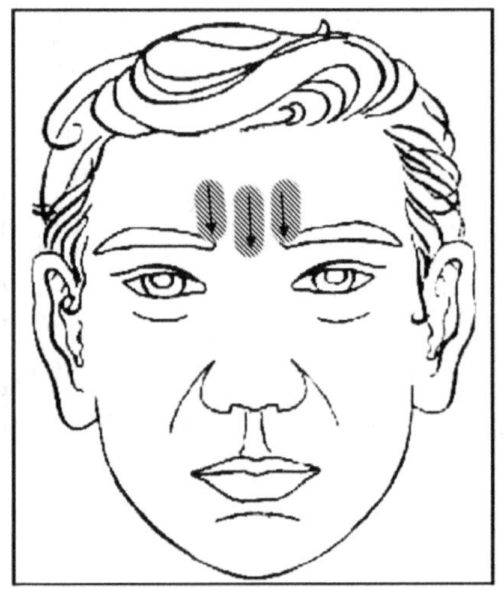

BURST OF HEAT

Massage from top to bottom the area between the two eyebrows, for about 30 seconds, then with the open hand, pass with the fingertips across the face, from top to bottom (you get results faster if you pass the roller toothed by Dien Chan).

Massage, with the index and the middle to V, placed horizontally, above and below the mouth. (see Uterus).

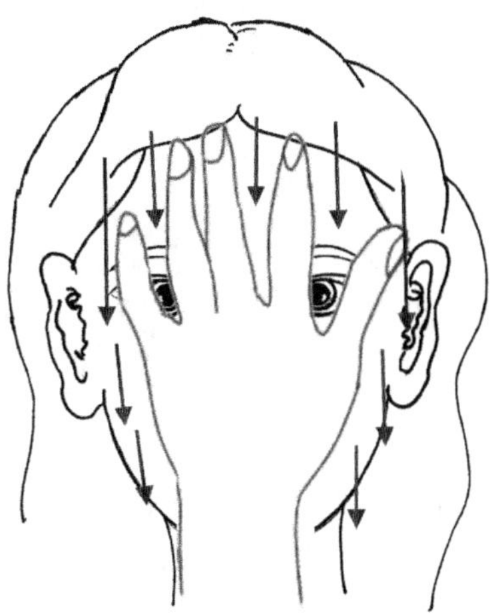

COLD

Press the point on the highest part of the chin curve for about 1-2 minutes (point 127); with V-shaped fingers, rub vigorously in front of and behind the ears; heat the auricles by rubbing them with your fingers or rubbing them with the palms of your hands.

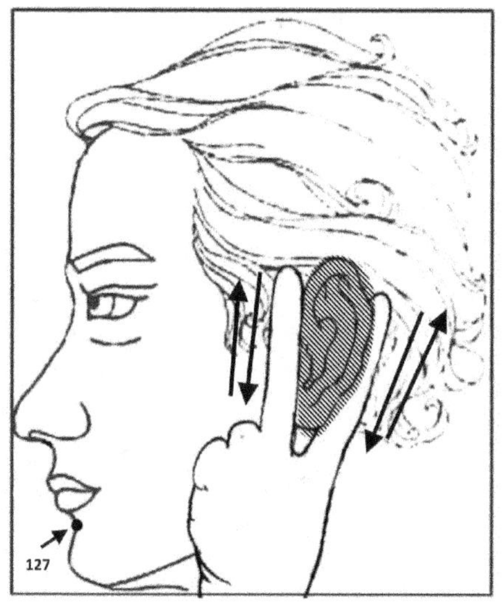

COLD (RUNNY NOSE)

With the V-shaped fingers, rub vigorously in front of and
behind the ears (see v. Cold) and, for the runny nose, press
the points in the middle of the nostril opening for about a
minute (item 287).

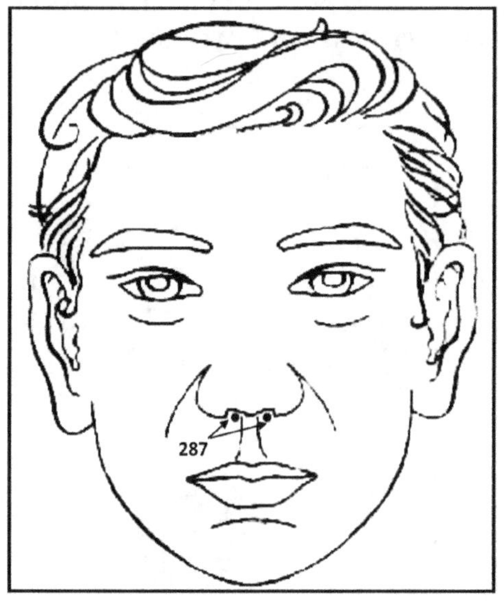

CONSTIPATION

Massage around the mouth, with the forefinger and the middle finger, on the upper lip, from right to left and then towards the center of the chin, descending vertically up to its extremity (like a large question mark around the mouth). Do it for about 30-50 times minimum, up to 200 times in severe cases.

BE CAREFUL DO NOT INVERT THE DIRECTION: THE SITUATION WOULD WORSEN!

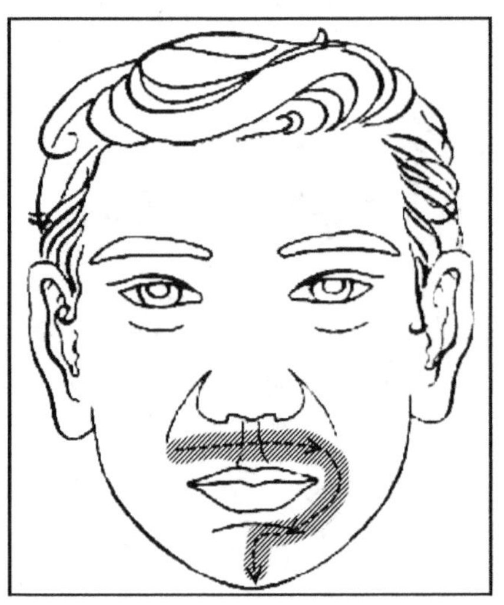

COUGH - INFLAMED THROAT

- Keeping your hands clenched in a fist, rub the inside of your wrists several times until you feel warm.
- Holding the left hand in a fist, warm up with the inside of the wrist (rubbing with one hand or using the heat of a hair dryer or a moxa).
- Grease the tip of a finger with some warm balm and rub the mouth of the ear canal a couple of times in order to leave a little balm in this area.
- Massage the area in front and behind the ear, from the bottom to the top and vice versa with the forefinger and middle V, until a certain warming of the area and of the whole body is felt.
- Heat the areas on the sides of the nose.

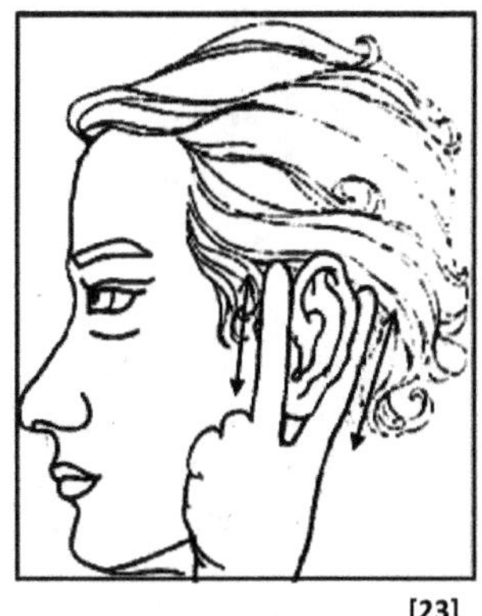
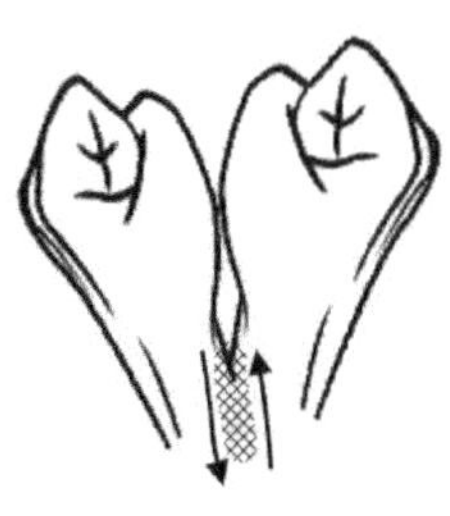

[23]

COUGH (PERSISTENT COUGH)

Press or massage downwards the central area between the two eyebrows. In addition, press the dimple between the two clavicles for about 1 minute.
If you have the heating balm available, grease the tip of a finger and pass the entrance of the ear canal with the greased finger, so as to leave a little balm in this area.

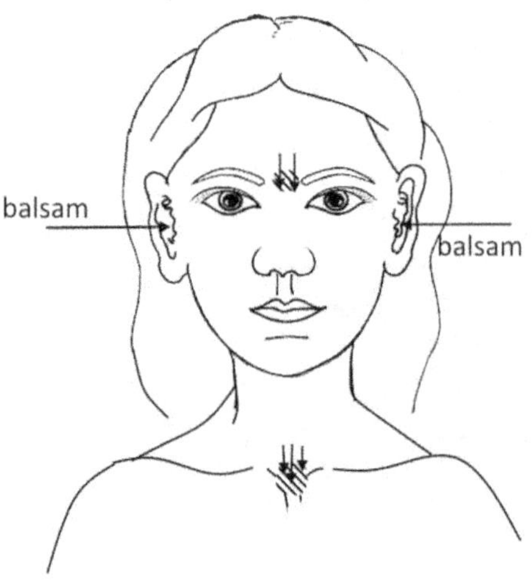

CRAMPS TO CALF MUSCLE

Beat the corresponding forearm 30-50 times with a hand in a fist.

Or quickly massage the dotted areas, as indicated.

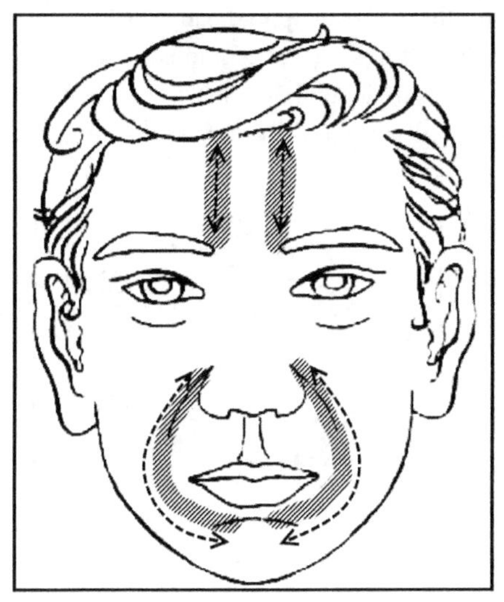

DIARRHEA

Rub the areas highlighted in the drawing with the fingertip for about 30 seconds, even with a little warming balm, if possible.

Repeat several times during the day, until you get good results.

For best results, you can apply heating patches on the same areas for about 2 hours (we recommend the Salonpas patch cut into squares of about 0.5-1 cm).

Remember to drink natural water with lemon, sugar and a pinch of salt.

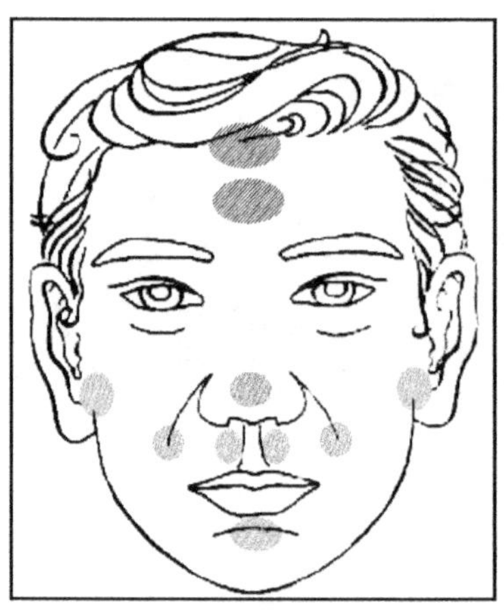

DROWSINESS

- Press point 19 for 30-60 seconds;
- Massage the ear pinnas up and down between two fingers
- Massage up and down the areas in front of and behind the ears, with the index and middle fingers placed in V.

WARNING: THIS MASSAGE CAN INCREASE BLOOD PRESSURE IN INDIVIDUALS SENSITIVE TO HYPERTENSION.

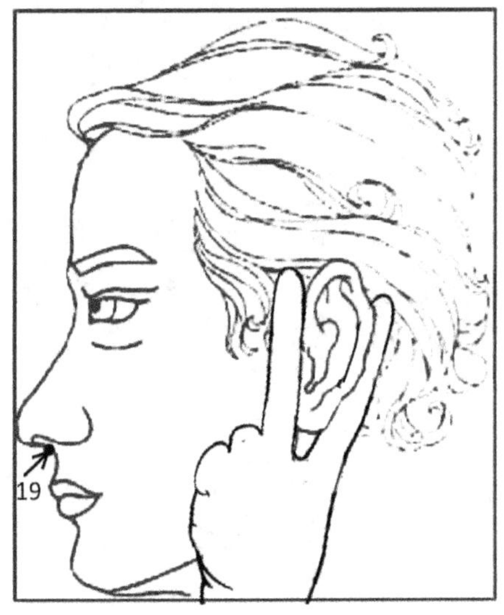

[27]

EPILEPSY CRISIS

Press the point 19 hard at the nape of the nose for one minute, then the highest point of the chin curve (point 127) and vigorously rub the ears of the epileptic.

After the crisis, massage the areas under the eyes and cheeks. This helps to rebalance the respiratory and cardiac activity of the subject.

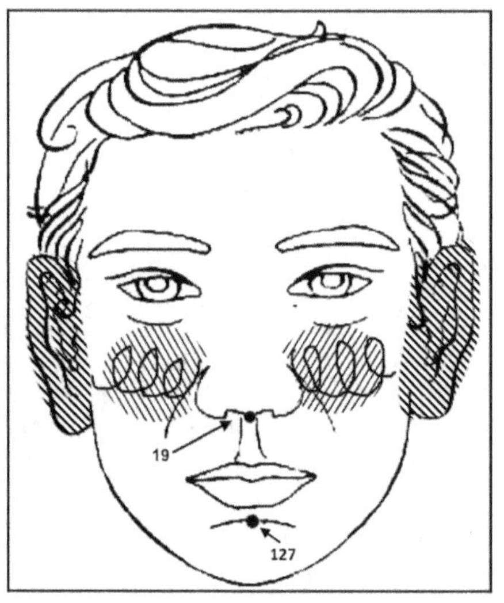

ERECTION

To stimulate erection, massage the nose from the bottom up for 1-2 minutes, with the middle on the nasal septum and the index and the ring finger on the sides, or massage the sides of the nose with the indexes, always from the bottom towards up.

WARNING: THIS MASSAGE CAN INCREASE BLOOD PRESSURE

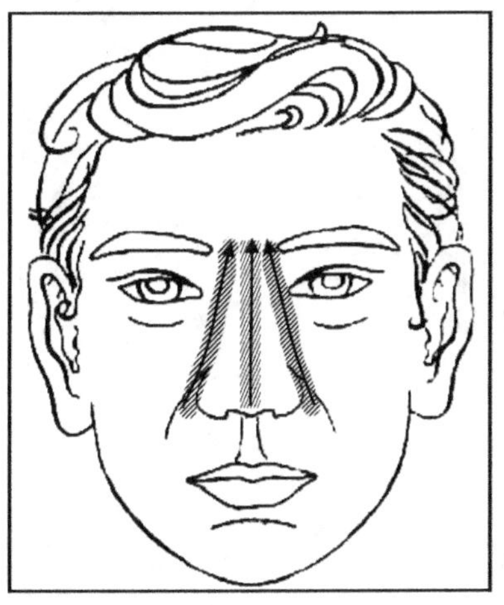

EYE - EXTRANEOUS BODY IN THE

Do not rub the eye because it could damage the capillaries; just stretch the tongue to the corner of the mouth for a few seconds: to the right to free the left eye and left to free the right eye. The eye will begin to water, taking away the foreign body.

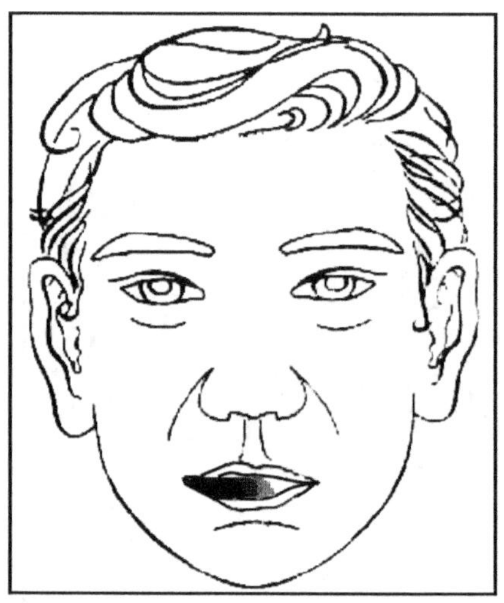

EYES - NERVOUS CONTRACTION

With the index finger, scrape the lower part of the beginning of the eyebrow of the pulling eye, for about 1 or 2 minutes (point 179).

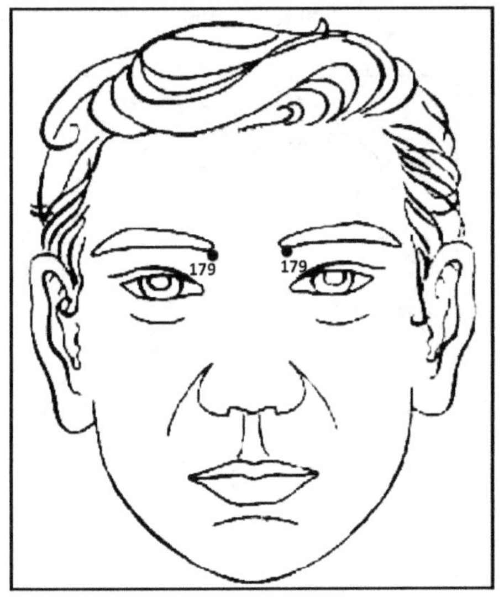

EYE BAGS

Apply a wet towel with hot water over the eyes and tap the fingertips around the same with the fingertips for about 3-5 minutes.

If it is possible, heat up with the hair dryer or moxa, or roll with a Yang roll of Dien Chan, the whole dark area, for a few minutes.

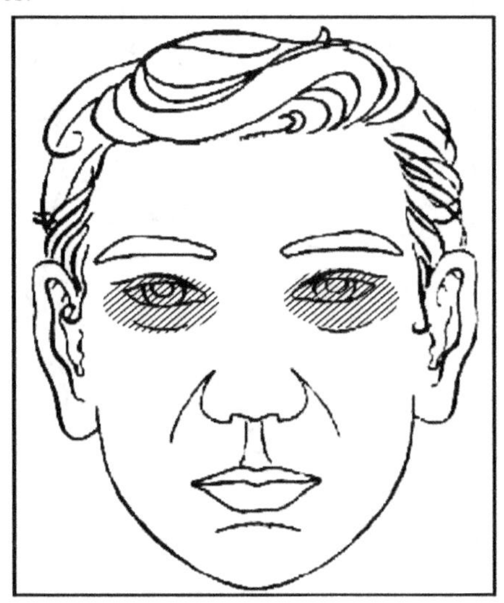

EYES (REDDENED EYES)

Stimulate with the knuckles of the fingers or with a DC instruments or some object with a rounded tip, the area of the palms of the hands immediately below the three middle fingers.

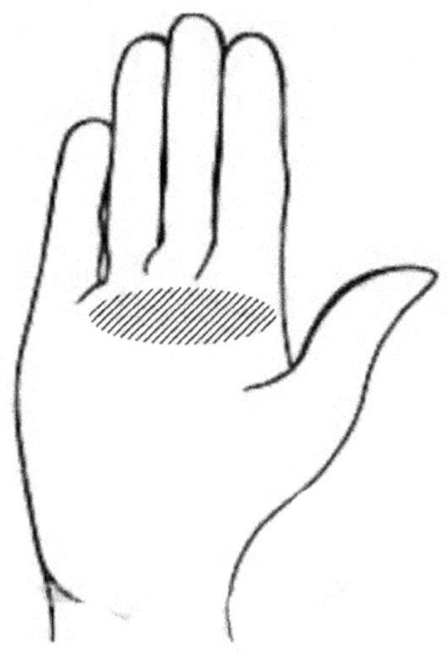

EYES (PAINFUL EYES)

With the indices, rub the upper area of the ear tunction, where there is point 16.

Pinch the side of the wrist between the index finger and thumb on the side of the little finger. If you feel a prickly pain, pinch 7 times.

Repeat all if the results are not satisfactory.

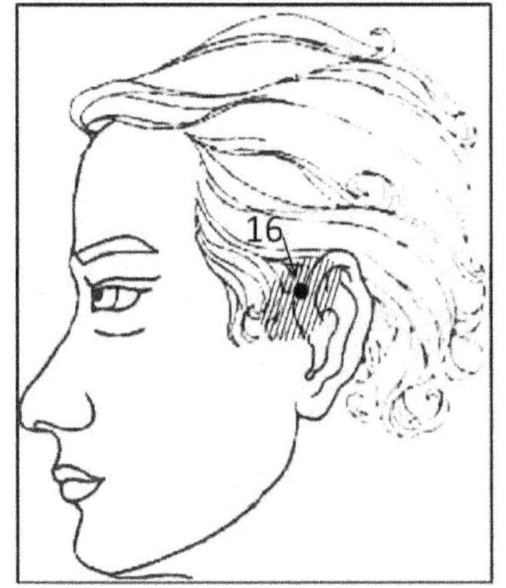

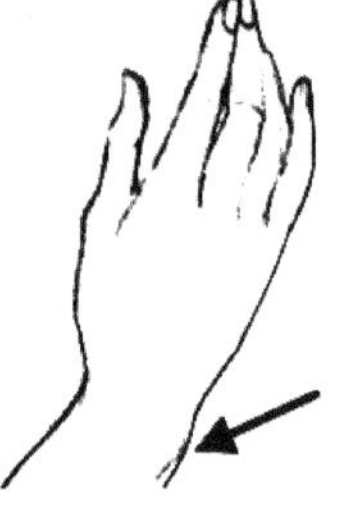

EYE – THAT CAN NOT CLOSE COMPLETELY

If an eye is unable to close completely, for example due to problems in the VII cranial nerve, heat with a hairdryer (or moxa) the opposite eye several times a day, each time about 2 or 3 minutes. Gradually the eye will close.

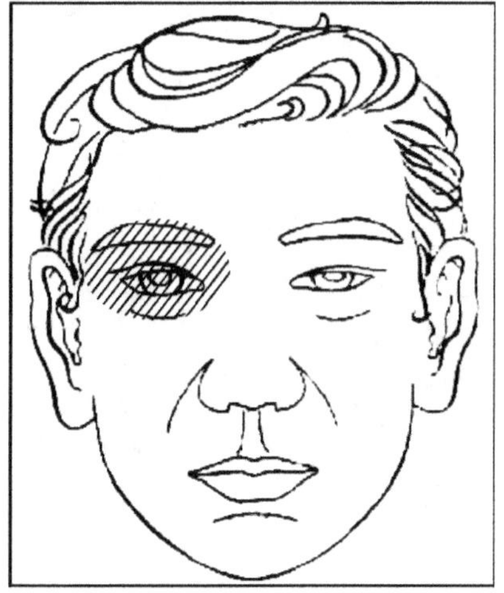

FACIAL PARALYSIS (V CRANIAL NERVE)

The main symptoms are pain and stiffness of the jaw.

Heat the outside of the thumb (massaging with the other thumb or using a hair dryer or moxa), from the nail towards the wrist. If the part of the affected face is right, the right thumb is stimulated, if the affected part is on the left, the left thumb is stimulated.

Remember to keep your hand open with the palm upward while moxing.

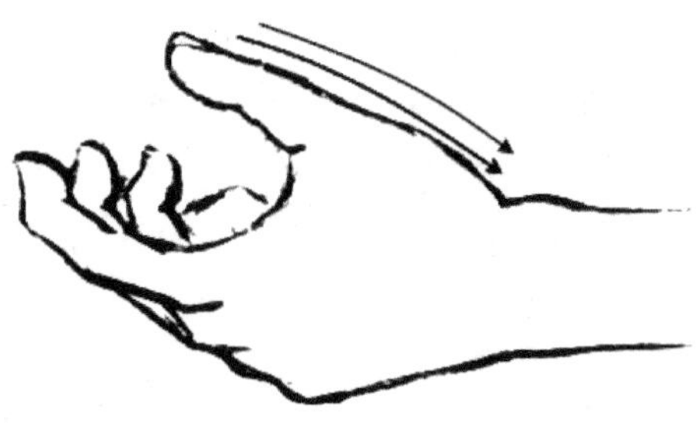

FACIAL PARALYSIS (VII CRANIAL NERVE)

Usually two symptoms are noticed: the eye does not close and the mouth is downwards, on the affected side.
Practice the following stimulations several times a day (3-4 vv), at least for 7-10 days before giving up.
- Warm up the "good" eye with moxa for a few minutes
- With your fingers or with the roller, pull or roll from the "falling" corner of the mouth towards the top of the ear.

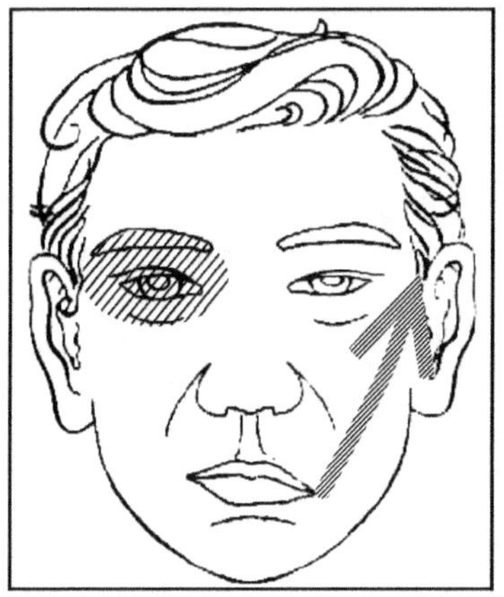

FAINTING

Hold on point 19 until the patient returns conscious. If this does not happen, press point 127 and 0 (zero) at the same time; at the same time massage your ears energetically or with a little balm. Continue keeping point 0 and the areas highlighted in the figure warm to get results faster.

(point 19 is at the base of the nose, you press it with your finger at about 45 °)

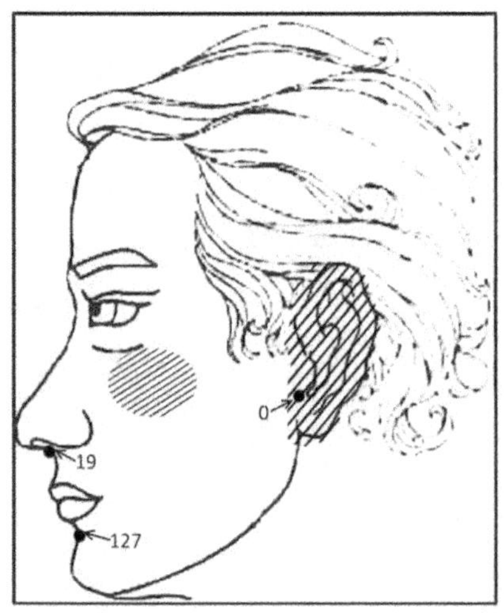

Wipe and press, even with a little warming balm if possible, the areas in the figure until the area is heated; alternatively heat the same areas with the hairdryer or moxa.

Repeat at least three times a day until good results are achieved.

To get results faster, avoid ice, cold water, orange juice, take a bath with cold water at night.

We recommend eating ginger, curcumin and hot food.

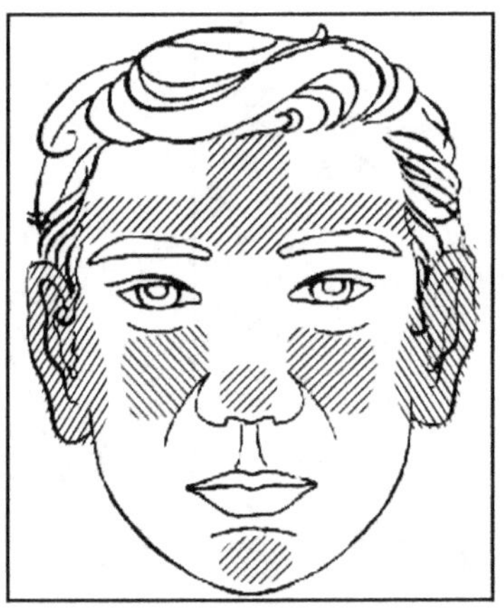

GASTRIC ACIDITY

Massage the two areas under the cheeks and the sides of the nose.

Holding your hand in a fist up, massage the forearm with your thumb, from top to bottom, where you feel more pain, insist more.

Repeat several times if necessary.

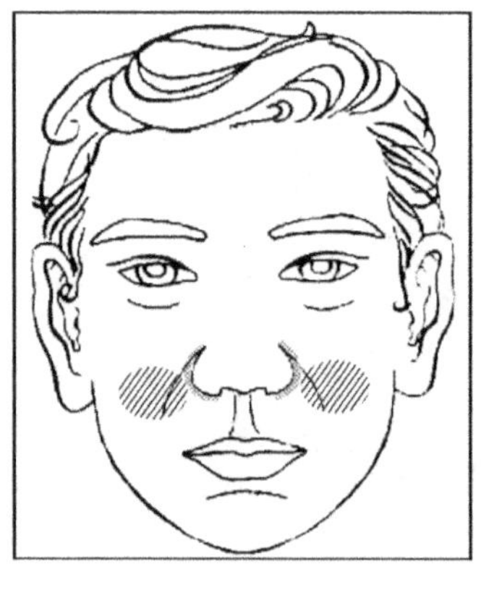

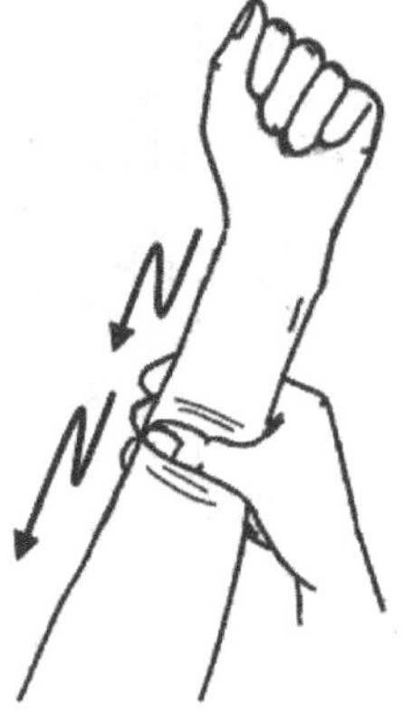

GLANS PAIN

Massage, pinching with the index and middle fingers, the tip of the nose for a few minutes or heat the same area with the hair dryer (or with the moxa) for about 1 minute.

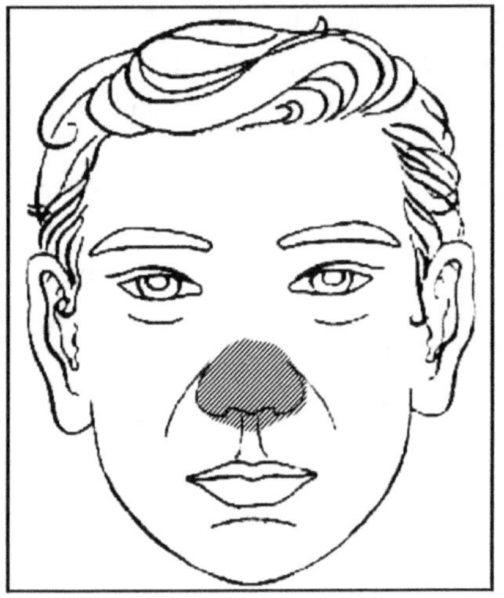

HEADACHE

According to the similarity theory of form, the hand clenched, pointing upwards, is the reflection of the head. You can then stimulate the fist to treat all types of headaches.

If the pain hits the right half of the head, mox the right side of the fist, if it hits the left half, mox the left side. If the pain is on the nape of the neck, mox the outer part above the wrist while if it is on the zenith, mox the knuckle of the middle finger.

If the pain is on the forehead, mox the folded part of the four fingers.

If the pain is on the temples, mox the side parts of the fist.

• Mox, in all these cases, means to heat up the affected area with moxa for about 1 or 2 minutes. In the absence of moxa, the hairdryer can also be used.

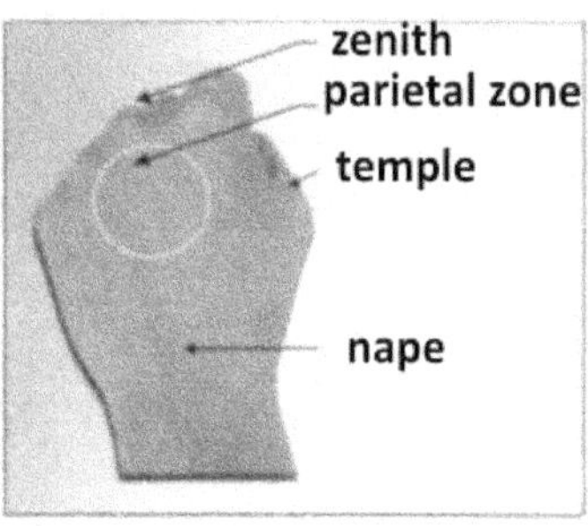

On the face you can stimulate the dotted areas with a pat, a pressure or a massage backwards.

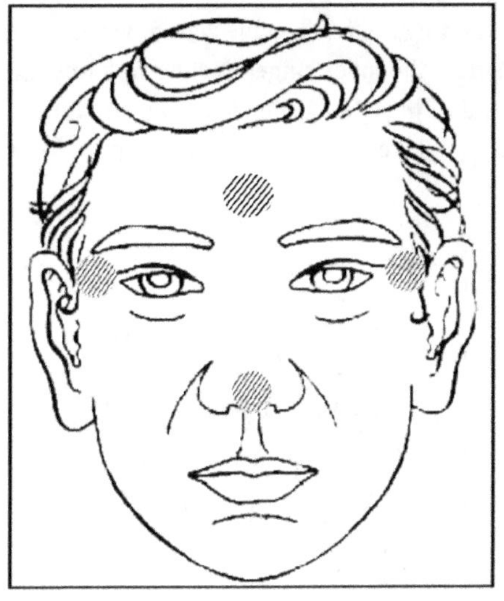

HEAT

Massage the whole face from the forehead to the chin, with the fingertips of the fingers, keeping the fingers open and slightly curved.

The middle finger passes on the central vertical, then the nasal septum, the index finger and the ring finger pass on the vertical of the eyes while the thumb and the little finger will massage the external parts, ending up on the chin

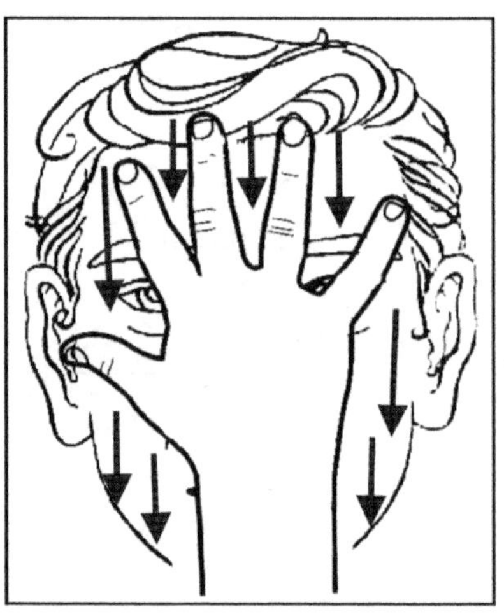

HEMORRHAGE

Press or wipe points 16, 61, 0, on the left side, for a few minutes; after which it is possible to apply small pieces (5 mm ^) of the Salonpas patch on them to prolong the treatment (the point 287 can also be added if the results are late in coming in. This point is in the middle of the opening of the nostrils).

This technique can be used for epistaxis, small cuts and can help in serious cases waiting for the arrival of the official first aid service.

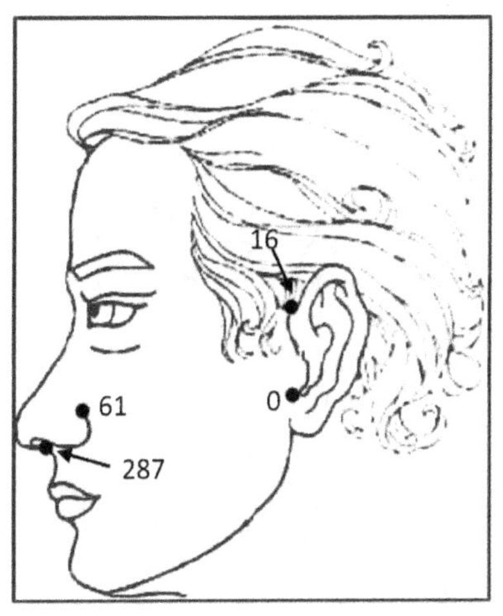

HEMORRHOIDS

Close the left hand in a fist, leaving a small opening in the center. With the thumb of the right hand, make a gesture as if to push something into the central opening. Repeat this movement for about two minutes (about 100 times) and check whether the discomfort has diminished.

Repeat the massage even two or three times a day, until the disorder has disappeared.

WARNING: IF IT IS NOT NECESSARY, DO NOT INSIST, BECAUSE THIS COULD LEAD TO CONSTIPATION.

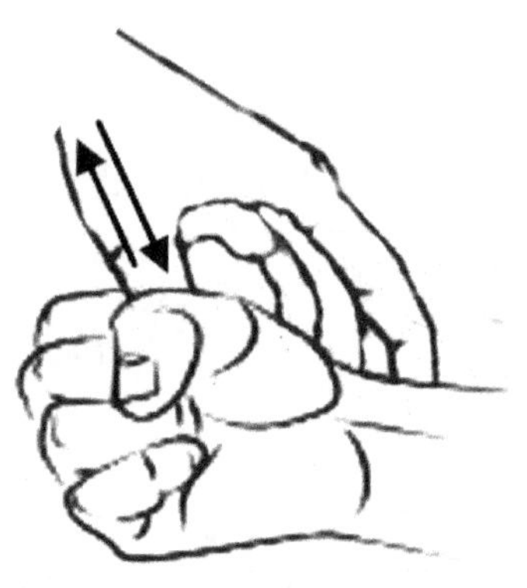

HICCUP

Try one of the following stimulations:

a) Using the index finger, tap the point between the eyebrows (points 26 and 312) about 15 times: point 26 has a calming effect and point 312 has a decongestant effect;

b) Massage the left side of the nose, from top to bottom, about 15 times with the index finger;

c) Approach the tips of the 4 fingers from the forefinger to the ring finger, scrape the scalp from the center of the hairline to the zenith of the head.

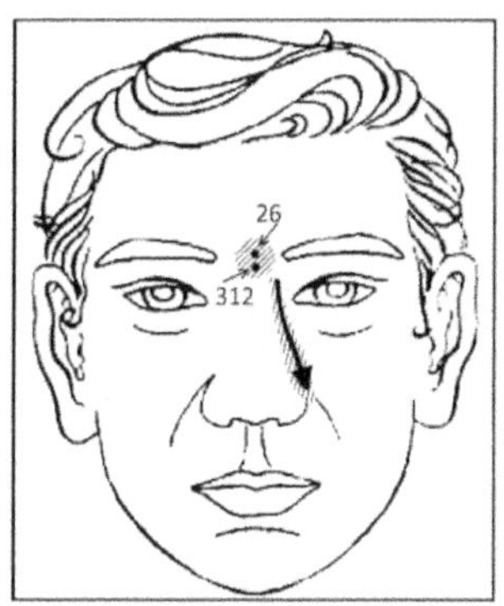

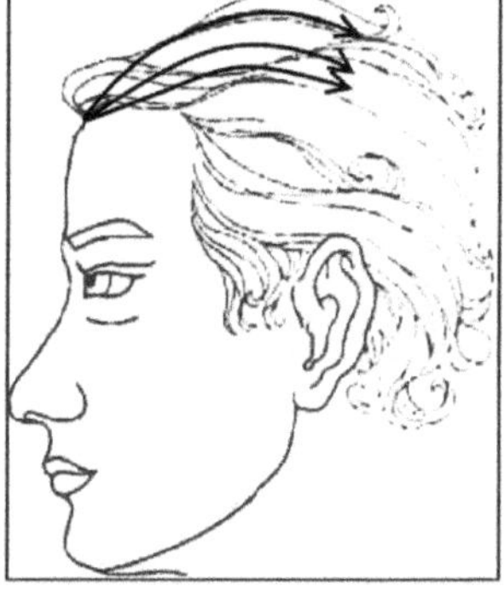

HIP PAIN

Massage the fold of the nostril, on the same side of the painful hip.

Or check the base of the two index and middle fingers positioned as inverted the V if there are painful pressure points. In this case, massage by pressing the painful point for about 30-60 seconds.

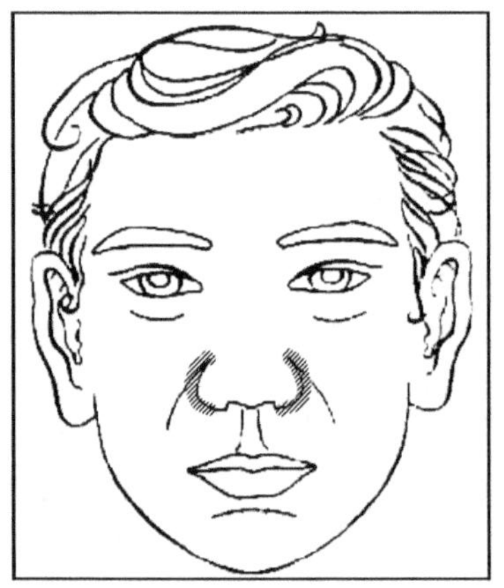

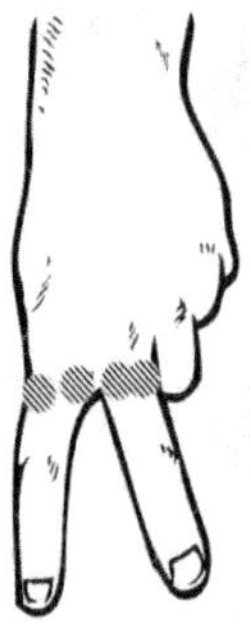

HYPERTENSION

Slowly massage the shaded areas according to the direction indicated by the arrows, approximately 30 times each area, and scrape the scalp from the forehead to the nape, always slowly, for about 2 minutes.
Start from the area between the two eyebrows.

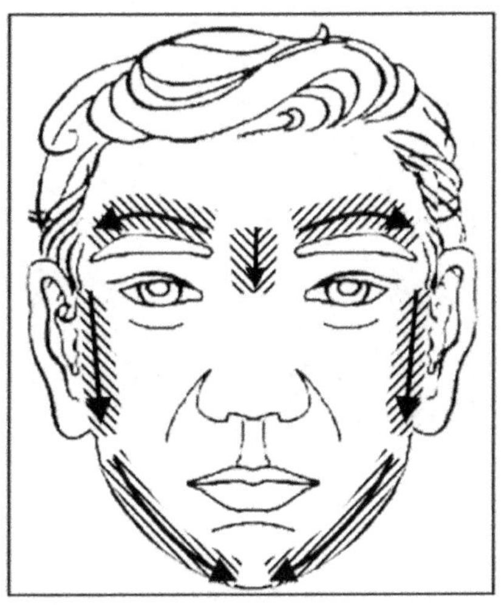

HYPOTENSION

Press point 19 for about 1 minute with a finger and repeat if it is not enough.

(point 19 is at the base of the nose, you must press it with your finger at about 45 °)

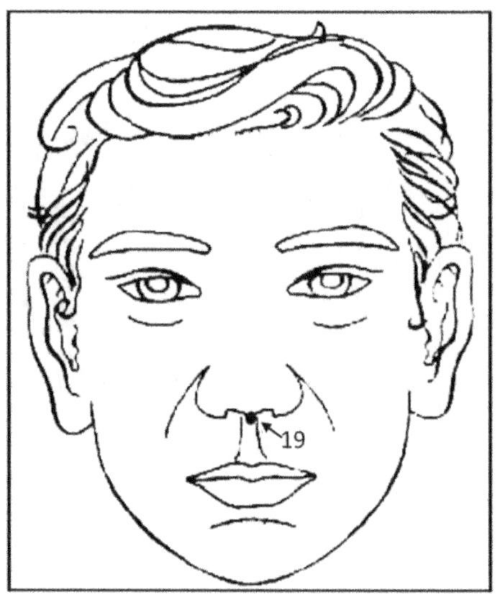

INSOMNIA

Before sleeping, rub your feet together or in your hands until they are warmed. If the feet are warm, the belly is warm and the whole body is warm. These are the conditions for a good sleep. Then, with the fingertip of the middle finger of the left hand, tap the centered point between the eyebrows approximately 1 or 2 minutes. The rhythm of the heart will calm and the mind will be relaxed.

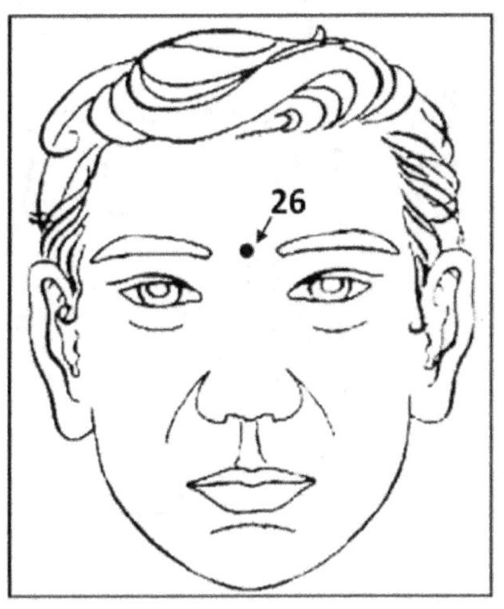

ITCH

Massage with a finger, from top to bottom, or tap, the area between the eyebrows (point 26) and the area under the right cheek, at the height of the base of the nose.

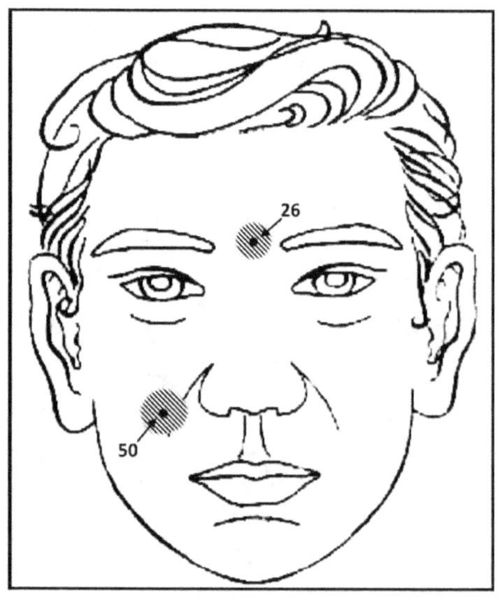

KNEE (ACHING KNEE)

Massage the dotted areas, alternatively massage the elbow from the same part of the sore knee, looking for the most painful point with the thumb and insist on it for about a minute or two, until the pain has passed almost completely.

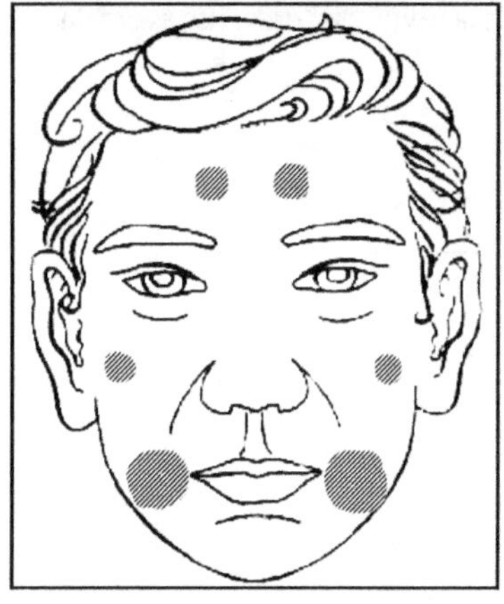

The expert crease of the thumb can also be massaged or heated with a hairdryer or moxa.

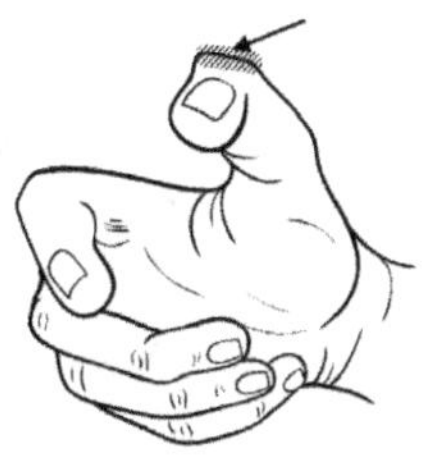

LACTIC ACID

Press the point between the nostrils for about a minute, as indicated by the representation of the nose seen from below.

This stimulation can also be done during physical activity, or immediately after this activity, in order to avoid lactic acid formation.

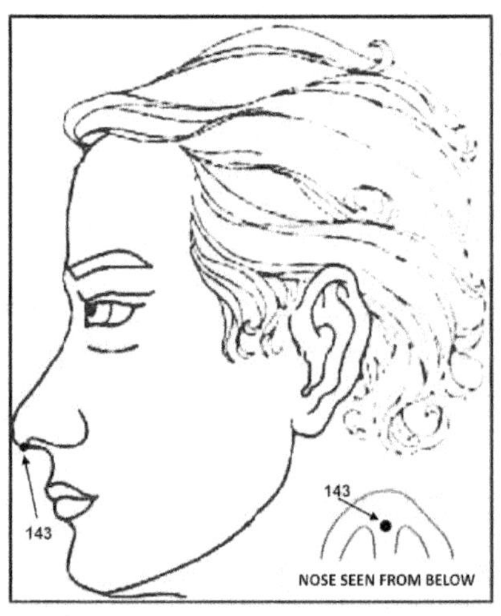

LEGS (HEAVY - PAINFUL)

Massage the dotted areas with fingertips for about 1-2 minutes. If you have a toothed roller, you can roll on the same areas for about 1-2 minutes.

Alternatively, or in addition, massage the two index and middle fingers, as an inverted V, taking them between the index and the middle, from the base towards the ends..

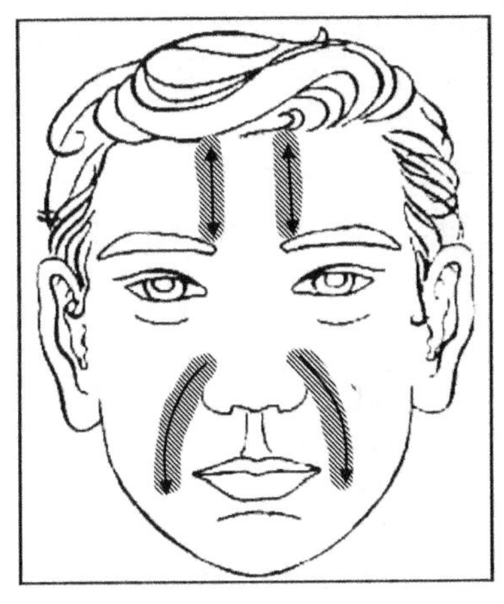
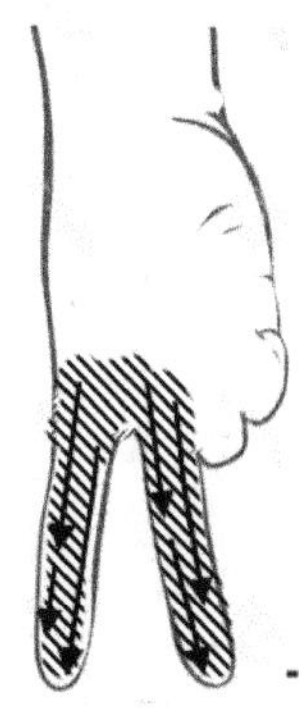

LUMBAGO

With the fingertip press and gently massage (or roll with
the Dien Chan toothed roller) the areas highlighted in the
figure. It can be a great help to apply some warming balm
on the same areas.

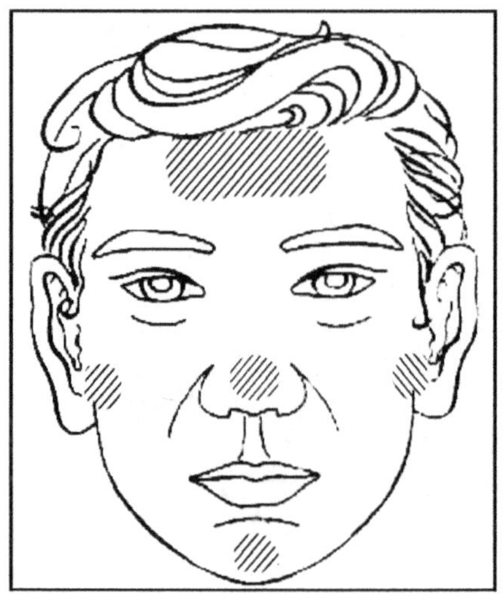

MEMORY – CONCENTRATION

Tap the fingertip of a hammer-bent finger with a fingertip for about 1-2 minutes at the center point of the forehead (item 103).

This massage helps to remember some information that we had stored and that at the moment does not want to come out.

It is very useful, done on a daily basis (even for only about thirty pats), to strengthen the memory of children, adults and the elderly.

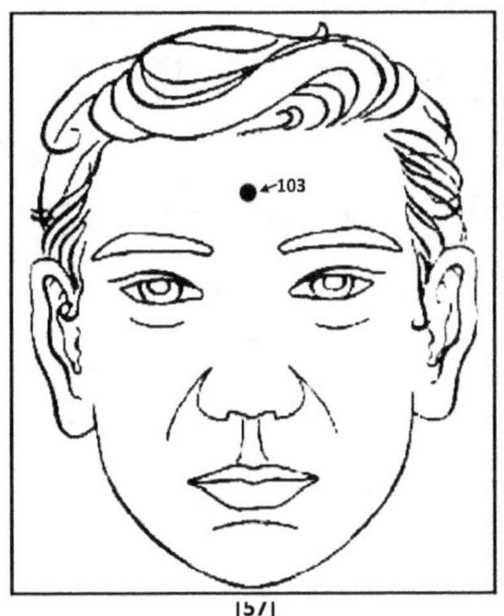

MIGRAINE

Massage the highlighted areas with the fingertip or cut 1 cm^ patches and apply them on the same areas. This treatment, if performed every day, can lead to lasting results.

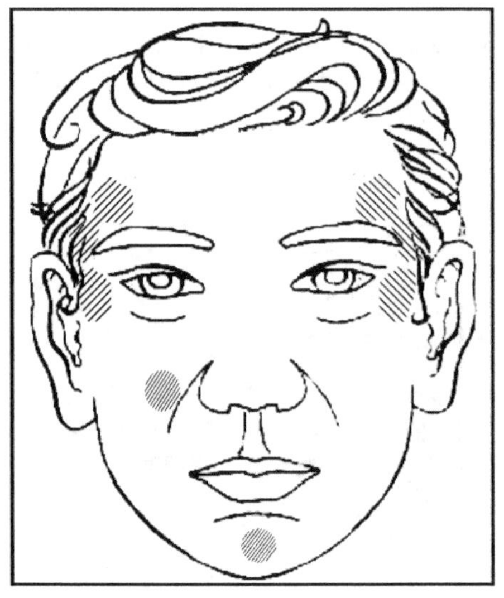

MESTRUATIONS (PAINFUL OR BLOCKED)

Practice these three stimulations:
- Immerse a towel in a basin of hot water, squeeze it and lace it over the eyes, putting a little pressure on the latter with the palms of the hands until the towel is no longer warm. Repeat the operation three times.
- Massage (or roll with the large double toothed yang roller), from the navel to the pubis until the stomach warms up, several times a day.
- Massaging above and below the mouth with the index and the middle, from right to left and vice versa, as shown in the drawing.
This last massage is also useful for menopausal disorders.

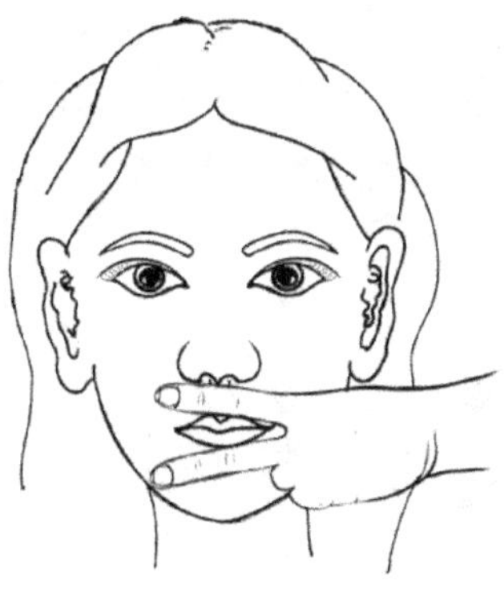

PANIC ATTACKS - ANXIETY - STRESS - IRRITABILITY

With the middle finger at the center of the forehead and the forefinger and ring fingers open, massage from top to bottom with a slow rhythm and a certain pressure, gathering the fingers towards the beginning of the nasal septum, as shown in the picture.

Repeat several times a day if the situation continues.

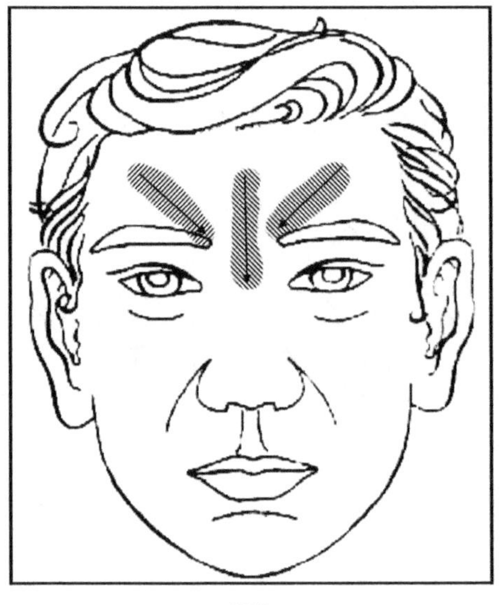

[60]

PAROTITIS

Press point 14 on the same side of the pain and swelling for about 30 seconds and heat the area in front of the lobe on the opposite side with moxa for about a few minutes. Repeat several times a day. the discomfort will pass in a few days.

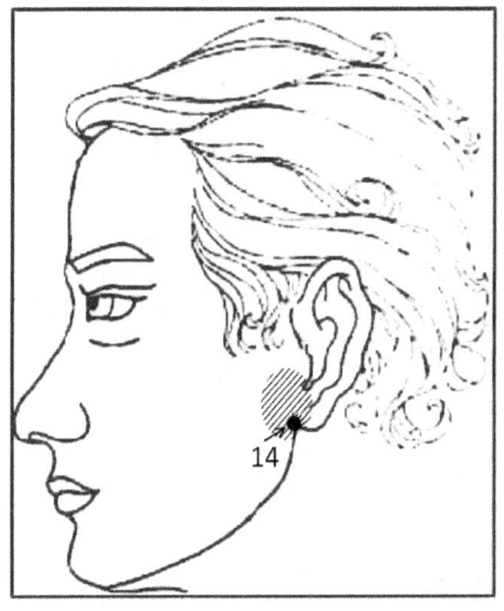

SCIATICA

Massage the scalp (the parts highlighted in the figure) with the fingers of the hands folded (or with the rake of Dien Chan). It is necessary to continue to massage until it is possible to lift or move the leg with ease (for 5-10 minutes).

This massage is to be repeated three times a day until the illness has completely disappeared.

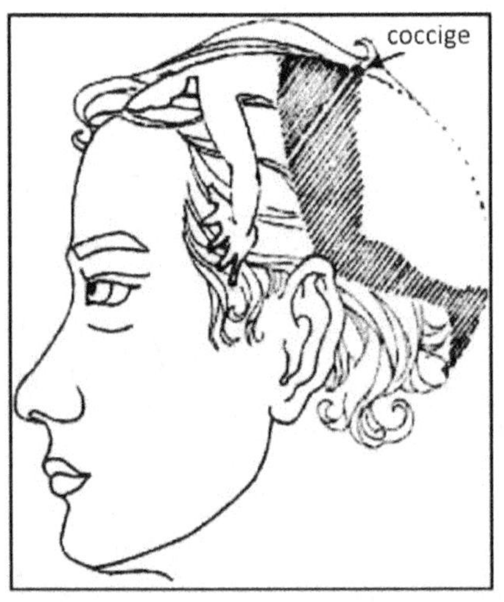

SEA SICKNESS

Press the center point between the nose and the upper lip (point 63) and point 0 in front of the lower part of the auricular nerve for approximately one minute.

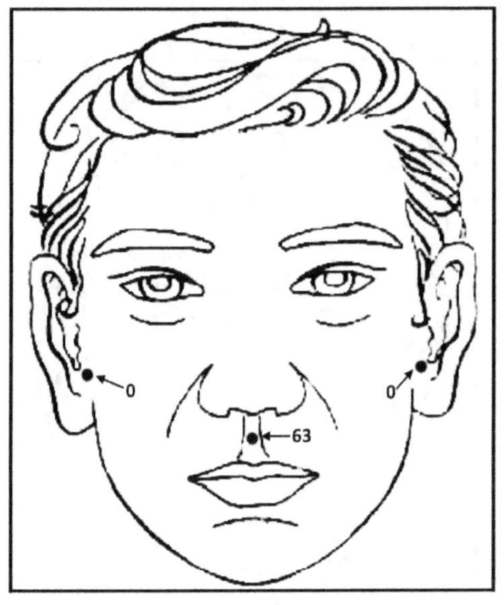

SHOULDER (PAINFUL SHOULDER) AND STIFFNESS OF THE NECK

Press and rub the areas highlighted in the figure with your finger. Continue until the pain sensation has disappeared or decreased by at least 50%. For severe cases, the massage is to be repeated three times a day.

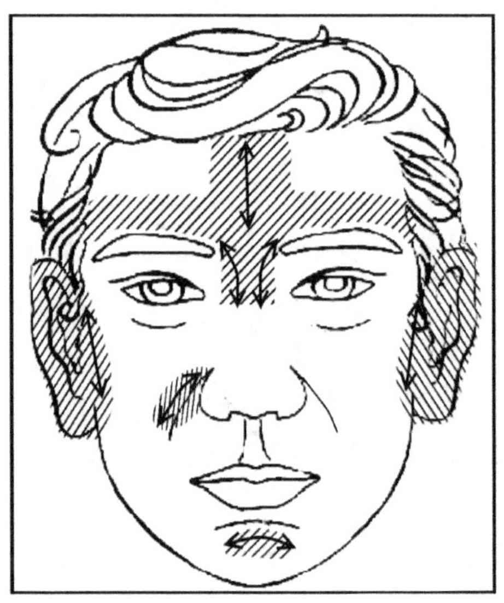

SHOULDER - PAIN TO THE ARTICULATION, DIFFICULTY TO RAISE THE ARM

Tap the forehead of the eyebrows with the fingertip of the forehead, on the side of the painful shoulder, for a few dozen times. The pain will decrease and the arm will raise. Repeat several times a day as long as the problem persists. (be sure that there are no fractures or injuries to nerves and / or tendons).

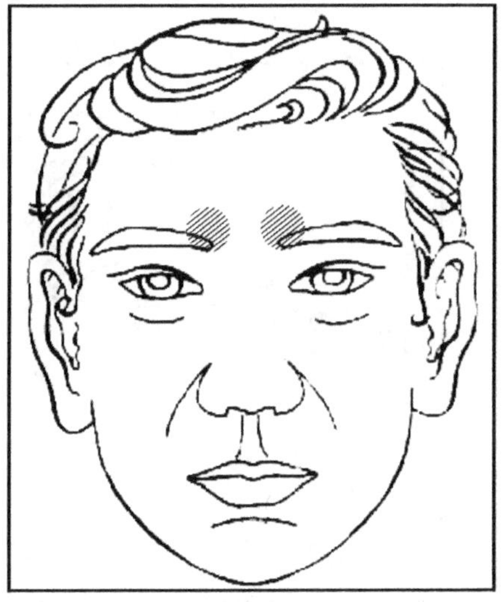

SNEEZES

Try one of the following stimulations:

- Massage from the center of the forehead (point 103) downwards the beginning of the nasal septum (the area of point 26), quickly and repeatedly

- Scratch point 287 (center of the opening of the nostrils) downwards with two fingers for about 1 minute.

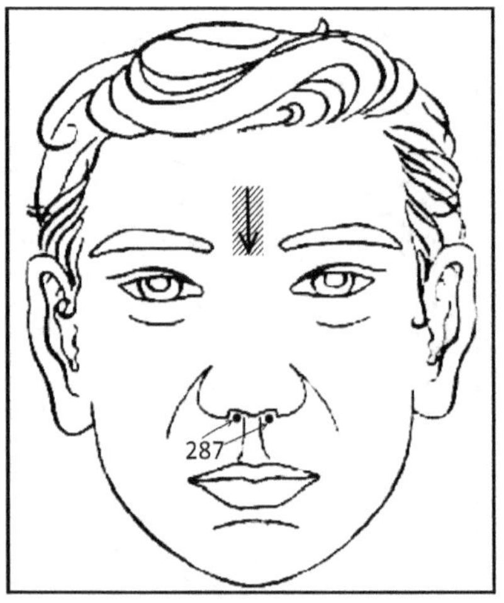

SNIVELER

Rub up and down until the dotted areas heat up, in front of the ears and above the central part of the eyebrows up to the middle of the forehead.

Faster results can be achieved by heating the aforementioned areas with moxa or a hairdryer.

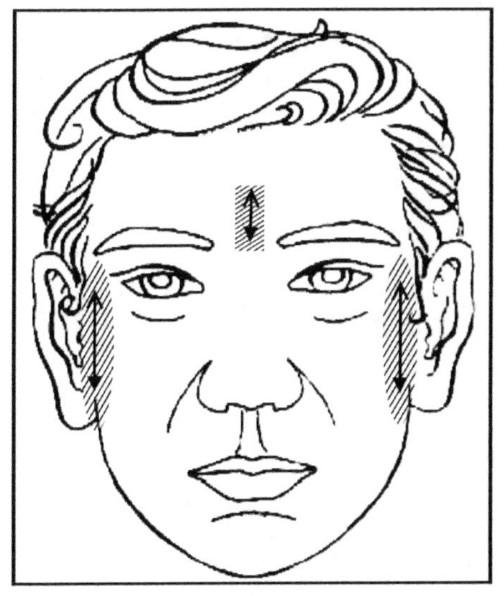

STOMACHACHE

It can pass quickly with one of the following stimulations:
- Heat the palms of the hands for about 10 minutes;
- Heat the soles of your feet for about 10 minutes with a hair dryer or rubbing them together or rubbing your feet with your hands;
- Heat the navel for a few minutes with the hair dryer or moxa, or apply a patch of about 2 cm ^ or put on some warming balm;
- Massage from right to left and vice versa the area under the nose and above the mouth, with the index finger above and the middle below. (**ATTENTION: TO BE AVOIDED IN CASE OF PREGNANCY**)

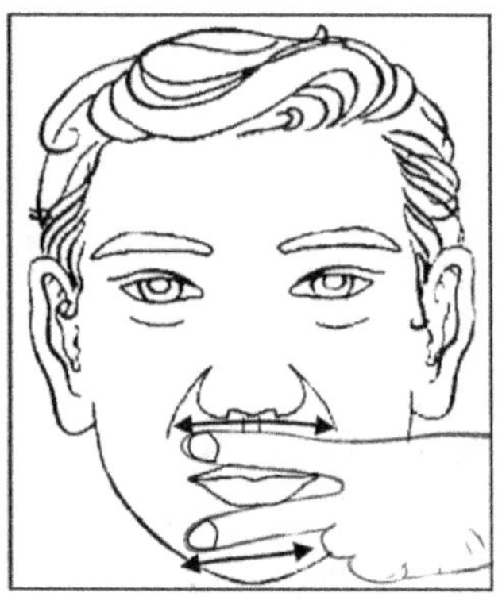

[68]

STOMACHACHE - DIGESTIVE DIFFICULTY

Heat the area around the navel for about 2-3 minutes with a massage or with a hair dryer or with moxa. Alternatively or in addition, massage with the fingers under the cheeks and the area above the upper lip (to be done away from the others because there will be air leaks ... or up or down, however not very elegant!).

This massage is useful even in the case of swollen belly

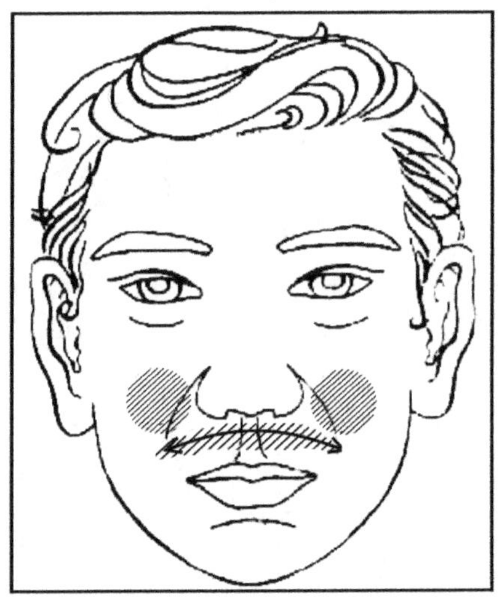

SUFFOCATION (EXTRANEOUS BODY IN THROAT)

This maneuver can be very useful for choking children with various objects in the mouth, or for fish bones and ossicles that stick into the throat and for cases of drowning.

Press step 19 for about 1-2 minutes. The foreign body will be thrown out, or, if very small, channeled into the esophagus.

(point 19 is at the base of the nose, you press it with your finger at about 45 °)

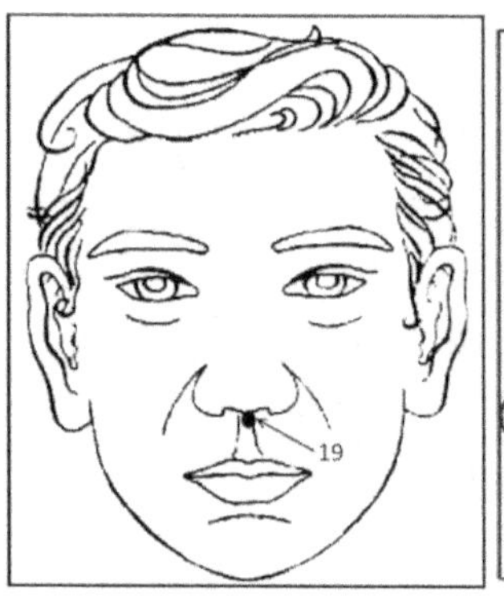

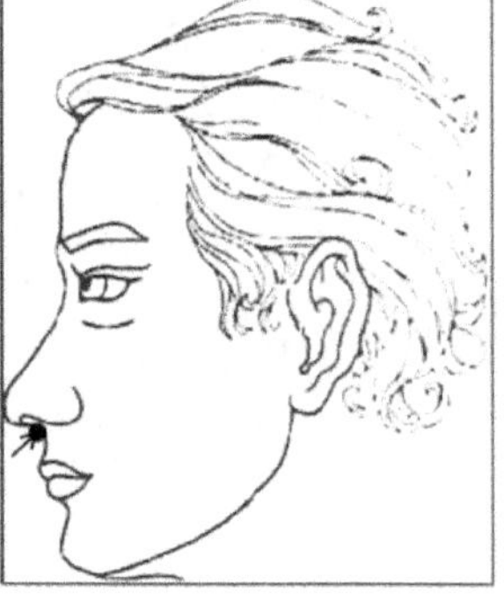

TACHYCARDIA

Press for one minute the following areas on both sides

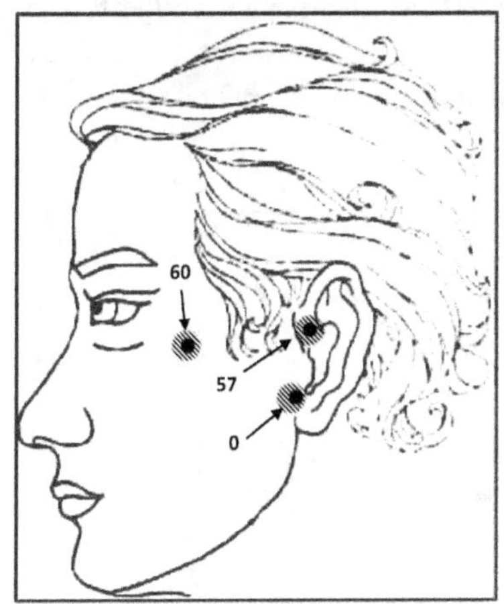

It is also useful to pinch the base of the little finger with your forefinger and thumb for a few seconds.

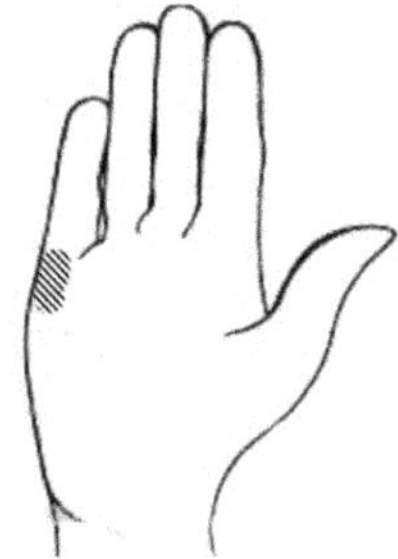

TEMPERATURE

Pass the brass roller, an ice cube wrapped in a cloth or piece of cold wet of cloth on the central vertical, from the top to the chin, then on the verticals that pass from the forehead over the eyes and go towards the chin. Do the same operation along the paravertebral, always from top to bottom.

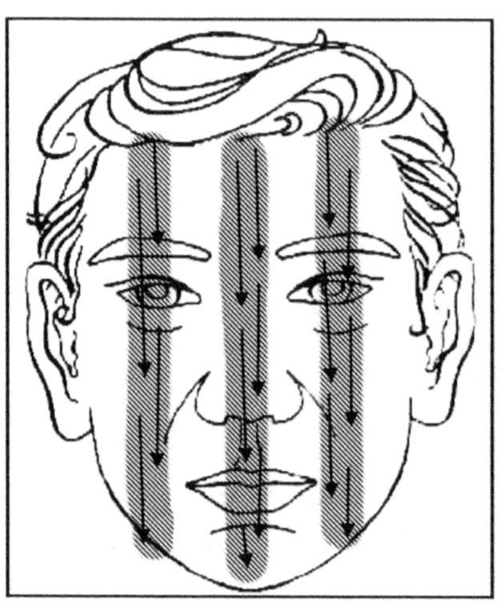

TONGUE (NUMBNESS OR STIFFENING)

Heat the thumb of the left hand for 1-2 minutes with the hair dryer (or moxa), then massage the same with the fingers for 1-2 minutes.

Tap the area in front of the ear lobes with a finger for 1-2 minutes.

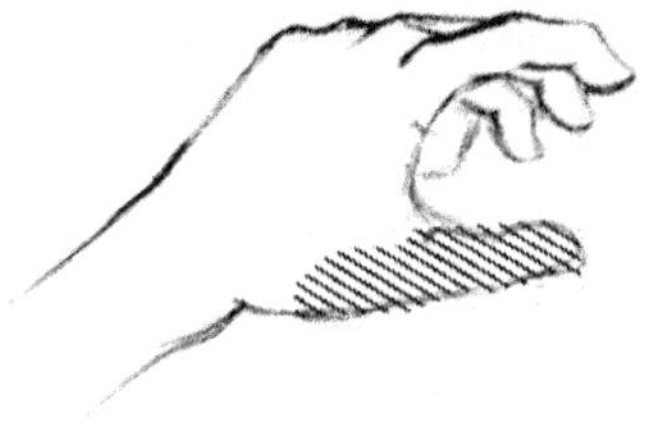

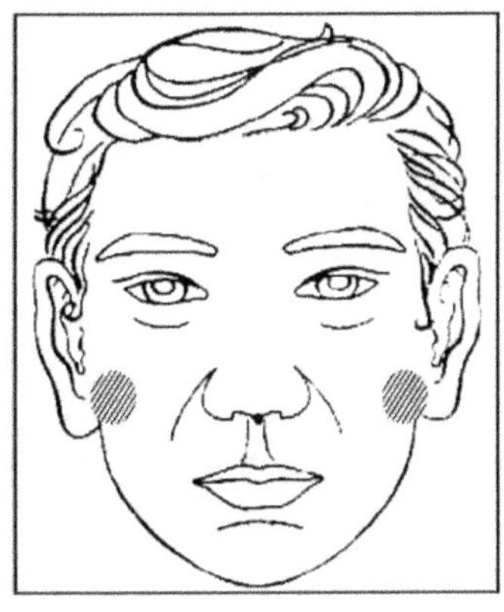

[73]

TOOTHACHE

Press or rub the areas highlighted in the figure with force. There will be good results in 5-10 minutes and it is possible to repeat it several times a day, until the pain has almost disappeared. You can also use heating patches (Salonpas) cut into small pieces (about 1 cm ^) and applied to the areas shown in the figure.

However, it is advisable to be seen by a dentist for a visit and more detailed information.

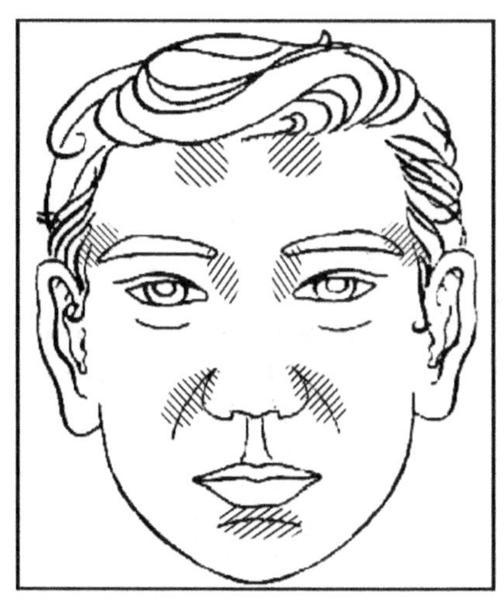

URINAL DIFFICULTIES

If you feel the stimulation, but you cannot urinate, massage gently the chin, from top to bottom several times, holding your thumb under the jaw and using the index horizontally.

This massage also helps children who urinate while sleeping or elderly who suffer from nicturia. It should be done about 15 minutes before going to bed.

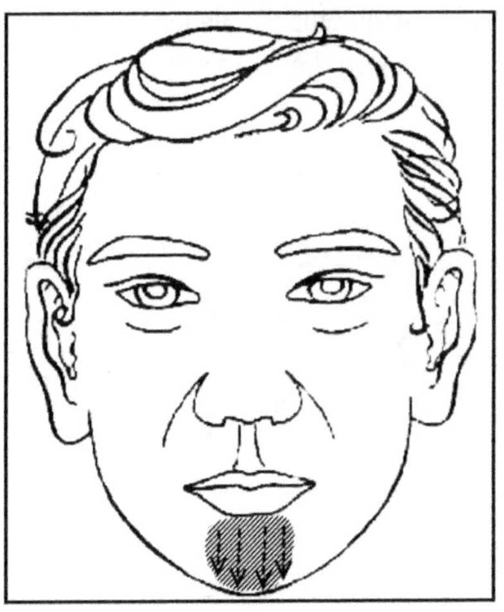

URINARY INCONTINENCE

If it is difficult to hold the urine, for any reason, with the thumb under the jaw and the index on the chin, press hard on the chin for 1 or 2 minutes, until the urination passes. However, it is necessary to look for the right place and "reopen the tap" with the opposite maneuver (see Urinary difficulties), otherwise our body cannot get rid of toxins.

This maneuver also helps for bladder prolapse, if performed every day and several times a day.

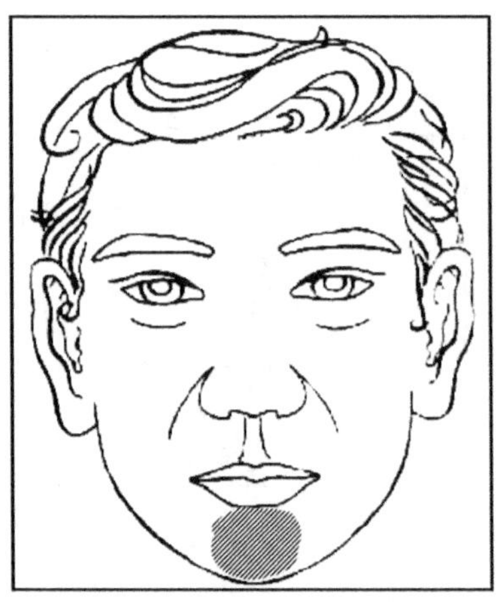

UTERUS (PAIN TO) - MENSTRUAL PAIN

Massage the central area under the nose, several times (about 1 minute and if it still needs repeating) or massage left and right, above and below the mouth, with the index and the middle placed horizontally.

ATTENTION: TO BE AVOIDED IN CASE OF PREGNANCY.

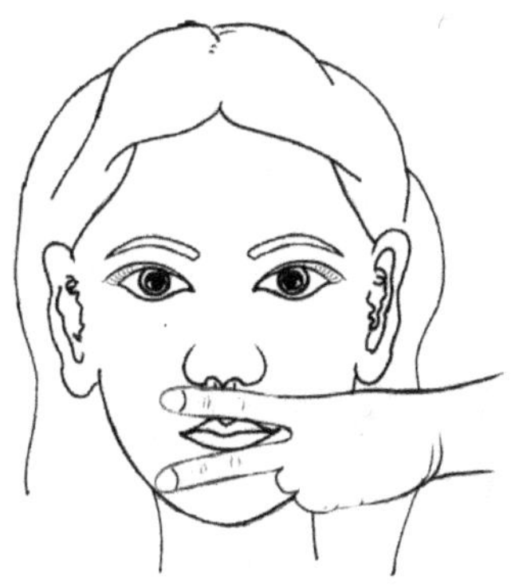

Press on the forearm in the area near the crease of the elbow, looking for a painful spot. Insist on the latter, with a tolerable pressure, for about 1-2 minutes.

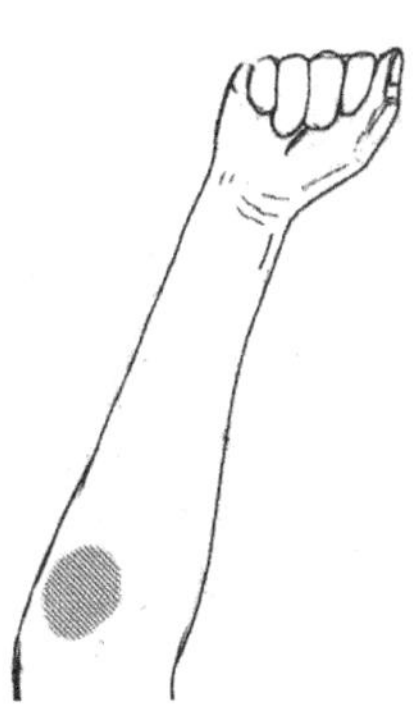

VAGINA (INFLAMATION, ITCHING)

By combining the tips of the index and thumb fingers, forming a slightly flattened circle, blow so as to refresh the inner part of these so positioned fingers. Alternatively, you can use a cube of ice or cold water (or a Dien Chan roll made of brass, with a gentle rhythm and little pressure), for about a minute. Repeat if necessary.

Another way to remove these hassles is to pass cold water, or an ice cube (or a Dien Chan roll made of brass) on the mouth, running from right to left and vice versa, for about 30-60 seconds and repeat if it is not yet enough.

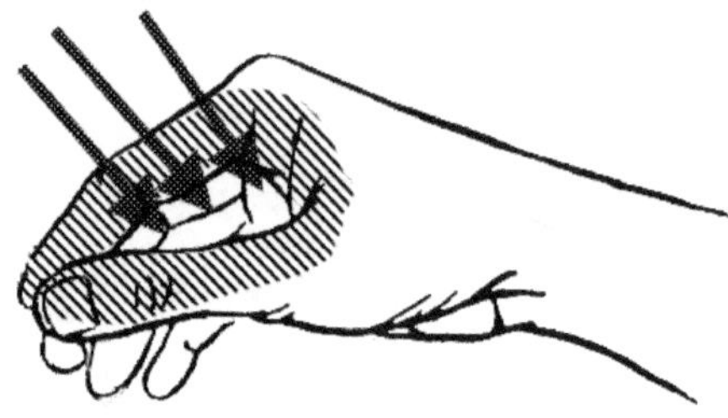

VAGINA - INCREASE SECRETION

Tap the center point just above the upper lip (point 53) until you feel a certain numbness (about 1 minute).

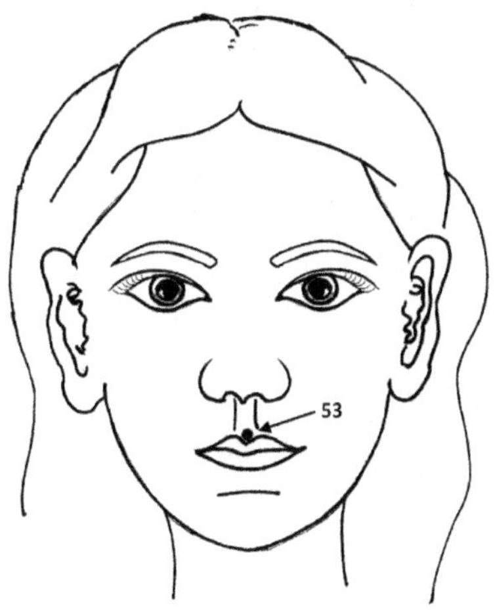

VOICE (LOWERED, DISAPPEARED, RASPING)

- With the open hand, massage the nape several times until it becomes all hot; you can also heat the same area with a hairdryer for 2-3 minutes.

- Strongly tap the area in front of the ear lobes for about 1-2 minutes (see figure) several times a day.

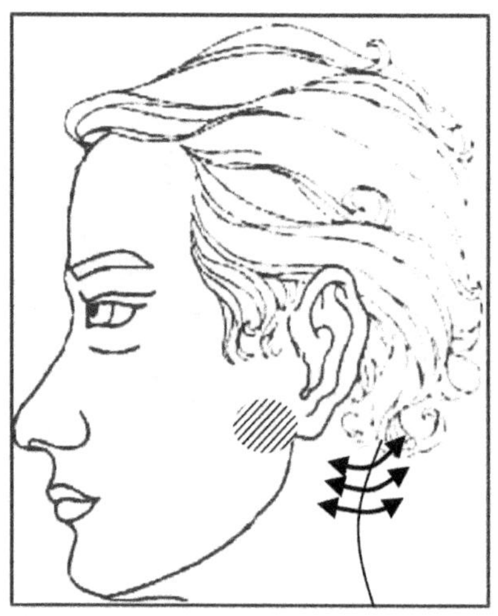

WRIST - DISTORTION OR PAIN

Rotate the healthy wrist for about 50-100 times and check if the situation has improved; carefully tap the end of the eyebrows with the index finger, on the same side of the painful wrist, for a few dozen times (to find the precise point corresponding to the wrist, point 100, press lightly under the tail of the eyebrows, where you feel a little dimple, there is the point to tap).

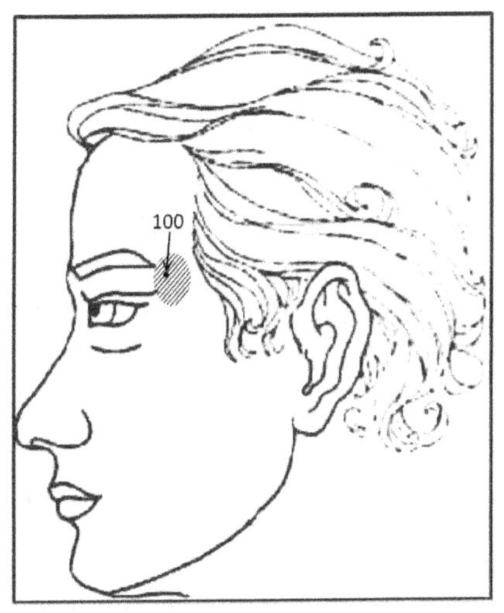

INDEX

TRUONG THI MY LE

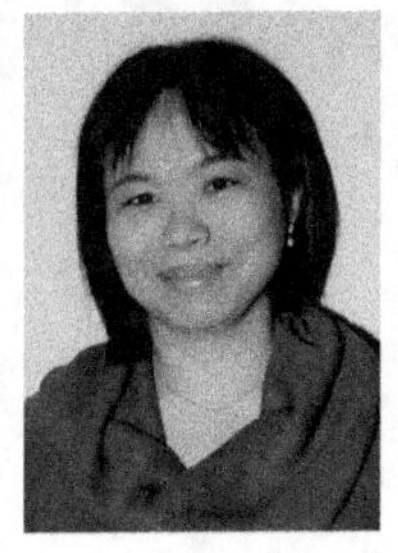

Born in Vietnam in 1972, she has been living in Italy since 1983. She learned the technique of facial reflexology from her brother Van Tri and attending via telematic the courses of prof. Bui Quoc Chau since 2012. In 2015 she attended the academy of prof Bui Quoc Chau in Vietnam and in the same year, on the occasion of the Dien Chan International Convention for the 35th birthday of the technique. In that occasion she received (together with his brother Van Tri), the recognition for the excellent work of divulgation in Italy and for the books of Dien Chan in Italian, elaborated on behalf of the founder.

In 2016, with his brother Tri, she organized the Master course in Vietnam with prof. Bui Quoc Chau translating its contents for 47 Italian reflexologists attendin the course. My Le currently works as supporting teacher for disabled students at a secondary school in Padua (Italy) and collaborates with the DIEN CHAN-BUI QUOC CHAU-ITALIA Association in the diffusion of Dien Chan - multi-faceted Vietnamese facial reflexology.

PROF BUI QUOC CHAU - TRUONG VAN TRI - TRUONG THI MY LE

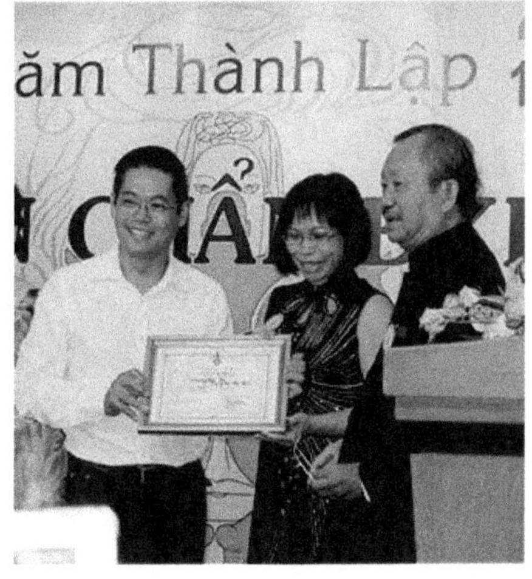

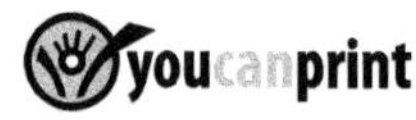

Finito di stampare nel mese di Aprile 2018
per conto di Youcanprint *Self-Publishing*